HIV-Positive

Debra Jarvis

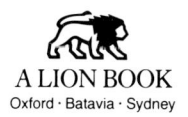

A LION BOOK
Oxford · Batavia · Sydney

Text copyright © 1990 Debra Jarvis
This edition copyright © 1990 Lion Publishing
Cover illustration copyright © 1990 Jeffrey R Busch

All rights reserved

Published by
Lion Publishing Corporation
1750 Hubbard Avenue, Batavia, Illinois 60510, USA
ISBN 0 7459 1820 4
Lion Publishing plc
Sandy Lane West, Littlemore, Oxford, England
ISBN 0 7459 1820 4
Albatross Books Pty Ltd
PO Box 320, Sutherland, NSW 2232, Australia
ISBN 0 7324 0129 1

First edition 1990

Library of Congress Cataloging-in-Publication Data
Jarvis. Debra
   HIV positive / Debra Jarvis. — 1st ed.
     p. cm.
   ISBN 0-7459-1820-4 : $2.50
   1. AIDS (Disease) — Psychological aspects. I. Title.
RC607.A26J38 1990
362.1'969792 — dc20 89-13070 CIP

British Library Cataloguing in Publication Data
Jarvis, Debra
   HIV positive: living with AIDS.
   1. Man. AIDS. Personal adjustment
   I. Title
   362.1'969792

   ISBN 0-7459-1820-4

Quotations from *The Holy Bible, New International Version*, copyright © 1978 New York International Bible Society

Printed and bound in Yugoslavia

CONTENTS

1	Denial	7
2	Anger	10
3	Blame	13
4	Forgiveness	16
5	Support	19
6	Peace	22
7	Balance	26
8	Relationships	29
9	Love	31
10	Healing	34
11	Death	38
12	Pain	41
13	Gricf	43
14	Hope	46

This book is dedicated to the Reverend Gwen Beighle who, through her work with the Multi-faith AIDS Project of Seattle, lives out Christ's call to love and service.

Preface

In 1985, as a fledgling hospital chaplain, I had my first contact with people with AIDS. I was struck by those I met — people who felt they deserved AIDS, people who felt totally helpless and hopeless about their medical treatment, people who suffered tremendous guilt about passing on the virus. Many were abandoned by their families and friends.

Four years later I began holding in-depth interviews with these people. Some of them lived in hospices, some with loved ones, some alone. We talked about many painful issues.

In the midst of what seemed like chaos to me, there emerged some people who were *living* with AIDS. Their lives focused on surviving, growing and beginning, not deteriorating, fading and ending. Instead of sitting in the darkness, they were walking in the light.

I have learned much from these people, and I have

included many of their words in this book. Some are still living; most are dead. All of them have taught me about the power of God's love.

Debra Jarvis

1
Denial

'I've heard about AIDS and I've read about it. Now they tell me that I have AIDS. I just can't believe it. I don't want to believe it. I can't accept it.'

What does it mean to be a person with AIDS?

You can make it mean what you want. You can choose to see yourself as dying. If you do, you will spend your time *dying* instead of living. Or you can choose to see yourself as a person *living* with AIDS. But you cannot deny that you have AIDS.

Denial paralyzes us. If we want to move forward with our lives, then we must move to a place of acceptance. We must move to a place where we accept ourselves and our emotions. And because we are human, we have painful emotions.

For some, being diagnosed with AIDS results in a feeling of grief and shock. Others feel numbness, almost a complete absence of feeling. Some are completely surprised; they never would have guessed they had the

AIDS virus. Others feel relieved at finally knowing, because for a long time they have silently suspected they had AIDS.

The implications of AIDS are overwhelming. You have just been told you have a terminal disease. Nobody gets AIDS and lives out a normal life span. Perhaps we once thought death belonged to old people and accident victims. Now we realize death belongs to everyone. Death belongs to *us*.

You may have friends who have died of AIDS and your grief for them is still fresh. Now you are faced with a similar path for yourself.

Or maybe you suddenly realize that you may have infected people you love. The pain of unknowingly hurting a loved one can be deep and intense. You find yourself reeling.

It is important to give yourself time to fully grasp what is happening. It may seem that you have no other choice but to accept your diagnosis. But at first you can also choose to deny it — you can try to go about your daily life as if everything is the same. Denial, however, is like putting a small bandage over a large incision. It may cover up things for a while, but it will not hold things together. Sooner or later, because of the changes in your health, you will have to face the fact that you have AIDS.

'At first I didn't believe the doctor. There she was, looking all serious and troubled. I wanted to laugh and say, "Well, it's not like I'm going to die or something." But then I thought, Wow, I am going to die. I didn't accept that right away. I kept the wild and crazy life-style I'd always had.

'But then I could see a direct connection between taking care of myself and feeling well. So I began eating better and taking my medicine. Ironically, my healthier life-style is what made my family ask me what was going on. When I could tell them I had been diagnosed HIV-positive, I realized I had finally accepted the diagnosis.'

2

Anger

'When I first heard my diagnosis I got really, really mad. Furious. I felt like somehow I shouldn't be, but I was angry and I didn't know what to do about it.'

It's not wrong to be angry about AIDS any more than it is to be angry about any other tragedy. And AIDS is definitely a tragedy. AIDS took us all by surprise. No one expected the number of deaths, or the kinds of deaths. No one expected the rapid rate of transmission.

There is no question that our anger is justified, and it is important that we express it. We can try to ignore it, but that won't work for long. Anger is like a big meal sitting in our stomachs. If there is something blocking the passage and we don't digest it, we get very ill.

So we must recognize our anger and digest it. We need to process it, deal with it, give it a voice. Talk to friends, scream in a pillow, beat on the bed. Get it out.

Dealing with anger does not mean we will never be angry again. Anger may well up in us every day. If so, we need to express it every day.

Anger itself is neither good nor bad. Its value is determined by what we do with it.

We can suppress our anger. We can keep it bottled up inside us until it finally eats us alive. We can lash out at people — people we love and people we don't even know. We can be angry and punish ourselves by not taking time to rest, eat well, maintain relationships. These are negative uses of anger.

There are also positive ways to deal with anger. We can use anger to fight disease, not just for ourselves, but for everyone. Anger can give us the energy we need to make changes in our lives.

Sometimes our anger about AIDS opens our eyes to other injustices of the world — hunger, racism, oppression. We can be part of the struggle to change those things.

'My first thought was that expressing my anger was extremely self-centered. What about all the other angry people in the world? What if everyone decided to express their anger?

'Then I learned that I didn't have to blow someone's head off to release my anger. I also learned that by venting my anger, I was better able to understand the anger of poor people, minorities, even other people who have AIDS. So expressing my anger actually made me less self-centered.

'It's like having a toothache — if you don't take care of it, all you can think about is your aching tooth. You can't think about anyone but yourself. Once you deal with it, you can get on with your life and be there for other people.'

3

Blame

'Sometimes I feel like a little kid — I am angry and want to find someone to blame for AIDS. Sometimes I feel like an adult and I simply want to find a clear-cut explanation. So far I have not been able to find either.'

Sometimes anger turns into blame. We want to find something or someone at whom to direct our anger, so we ask 'Why?' and demand an explanation.

It's hard for us to understand that ultimately there is no one thing or person whom we can blame. It's true that, for some, life-styles have contributed to increasing the chances of getting AIDS. For others, AIDS has entered their lives in a completely unexpected way.

We would like to make sense of it all — to explain. But we can't explain the presence of AIDS in the world any more than we can explain the presence of cancer or heart disease. AIDS is *not* punishment by God. It is not a question of who deserves AIDS. Nobody deserves AIDS!

We cannot satisfactorily explain why God has allowed *any* disease. Trying to use human reason to understand God's ways will get us nowhere. There is no easy answer.

It's hard for us to accept that we don't know the reason for everything. Two thousand years ago, people were asking the same questions. The gospel writer John tells us that Jesus met a man who had been blind since birth:

> His disciples asked him, "Rabbi, who sinned, this man or his parents, that he was born blind?"
>
> "Neither this man nor his parents sinned," said Jesus.

Then Jesus healed the man. He did not try to assign blame. Jesus was interested in healing and loving, not blaming.

Once we can let go of our need to explain everything, we are free to pursue healing and loving.

> *'At first I made a list of all the things in my life that I thought might have given me AIDS. I don't mean logical things — I was writing down stuff like "Age ten: destroyed an entire ant hill." I wanted to add everything up and see if the total equaled AIDS. It didn't.*
>
> *'It was hard for me to realize that life doesn't add up like a mathematical equation. But most people still run around with that idea*

*in their heads. When somebody asks me how
I contracted AIDS, I know that they've missed
the point. I know they're thinking if I did
this or that, then I deserved it. But that is not
how life works.'*

4
Forgiveness

'AIDS has forced me to stop and take a look at my life. I am so ashamed of some of the things I have done, the way I have lived, the people I have hurt. I can't see how God can forgive me. I feel so guilty.'

Everyone is guilty. All of us have said and done things we are ashamed of. So we all know that guilt and shame cause a serious sickness of the soul. But there is a cure, a way to find relief.

First, we have to admit to ourselves all those things we have been trying to hide from ourselves and others. We need to bring out in the open everything we feel guilty about. Then we can ask for forgiveness from God and from the people we've hurt.

After looking at our lives, it may be hard to believe that God would forgive us. The Old Testament prophet Nehemiah tells us that God is 'a forgiving God, gracious and compassionate, slow to anger and abounding in love' — but we may not know anybody who is remotely like that. So it may be hard to understand how forgiving God is. Think of the most forgiving person you know. Now multiply that person's ability to forgive by one billion, and you get some idea of how forgiving God is.

Not only are our sins forgiven, they are forgotten. God wipes the slate clean and gives us a new start, a second chance. The prophet Isaiah tells us:

'Though your sins are like scarlet, they will be as white as snow; though they are red as crimson, they will be like wool.'

It's important to confess our wrongdoing and deal with our guilt. If we don't, we either try to blame others or we start an endless cycle of blaming ourselves. Once we realize God forgives, we can forgive ourselves and get on with our lives.

Still, accepting that we are forgiven can be very difficult. We want to hang on to our guilt. Whether we recognize it or not, hanging on to our guilt keeps us from moving forward. Sometimes it's easier to stay in the familiar misery of guilt than to move out to an unfamiliar place of forgiveness.

It is our fear of the unknown. We are afraid to move on because we don't know what the journey holds for us. And it is so hard to believe that God really will accept us no matter what we have done.

But we *can* know that forgiveness is real, because God, in Jesus Christ, came to our world to be with us. Jesus stands beside us in our pain, our grief, our fear, our guilt. Jesus also suffered and died — he knows what it is like.

We know God will forgive, because we have seen his love in Jesus.

When Jesus healed a paralyzed man, he said to him, 'Take heart, son; your sins are forgiven . . . . Get up, take your mat and go home.' The man got up and went home.

Like the paralytic, once we accept forgiveness, we can get up, take our mats and continue on our journeys.

AIDS forces us to look at how we've lived our lives. Some of us have chosen to see AIDS as an opportunity to make changes in our lives, to let God transform us and make us new people.

'For a long time it was easier just to wallow in my own self-pity and guilt. In some kind of sick way I actually enjoyed feeling like everybody hated me. You know, I sort of took pride in being the saddest person in the world, because not only did I have AIDS, but everybody was mad at me.

'Then I had a friend who said she had been praying for me. She had been praying that I would know God's forgiveness. Hearing somebody say God forgives me blew my mind. Then I had no reason to feel sorry for myself or to feel guilty. Then I was able to resolve the past with everybody else. My guilt was like a hundred-pound weight on my leg.'

5

Support

***'I** want to deal with my anger and shame. **I** want to change my life, but I just can't do it alone.'*

Nobody has to do it alone. The paralyzed man was brought by his friends to be healed by Jesus. He did not come alone.

If you have been rejected by families and friends, it's natural to feel alone. Now you have to create a new family for yourself. You have to look for environments of trust and support. There *are* people who will care, listen and comfort.

Yet because of previous rejection, many are afraid to ask for help. So they sit — in fear and in need.

But we all have a choice.

Instead of waiting for the phone to ring, we can choose to pick it up and call someone. Instead of looking at one another in fear, we can choose to see ourselves reflected in one another. Instead of hating, we can choose to love. As long as we remember that we have choices, we know that we are neither victims nor helpless.

Having AIDS does not mean that you are reduced to a pitiful human being who has nothing to give. You can still love and laugh and give of yourself. The most valuable gifts come from the heart: a tender word, a touch, a smile, a tear.

AIDS has made many of us realize that all of humanity is interconnected. We are woven like threads through a beautiful piece of fabric. God loves every fiber of each thread. When we hurt one another, we hurt ourselves and we hurt God. When we help one another, we help ourselves and we help God.

God, others, ourselves. This is what Jesus was talking about when he was asked which were the most important commandments. He answered:

'Love the Lord your God with all your heart and with all your soul and with all your mind and with all your strength. And love your neighbor as yourself.'

'I was really depressed because my family had kicked me out. My father gave me five dollars and told me never to come home again. I thought that little incident would kill me before AIDS did. I figured if my family cast me out, strangers certainly wouldn't want me.

'I got the surprise of my life when people in the clinic, people at a nearby church, people in my apartment building actually became my friends. If you had told me that would happen, I

never would have believed it. So it was as if I got a whole new family. Being part of a family means giving too, and so giving to others got me out of myself. It's easy to be super self-centered when you have AIDS. But caring about other people helped me.'

6
Peace

'It's funny — even though my head wants to feel peace and acceptance, in my heart I feel anxious and angry. I can talk all day and all night to my friends, but even they can't help.'

There is a place in our hearts that can be filled only by God. Therapy, counseling and all the friends in the world cannot fill this spot. Only God can, and our task is to invite God into our lives.

We have not been abandoned. God is always with us to love us, comfort us and fill us with peace. Many of the Psalms are comforting reminders of God's presence and goodness.

The psalmist writes:

'O Lord, you have searched me
 and you know me.
You know when I sit and when I rise;

> you perceive my thoughts from afar.
> You discern my going out and my lying down;
> you are familiar with all my ways.
> Before a word is on my tongue
> you know it completely, O Lord.
>
> You hem me in — behind and before;
> you have laid your hand upon me.
> Such knowledge is too wonderful for me,
> too lofty for me to attain.
>
> Where can I go from your Spirit?
> Where can I flee from your presence?
> If I go up to the heavens, you are there;
> if I make my bed in the depths, you are there.
> If I rise on the wings of the dawn,
> if I settle on the far side of sea,
> even there your hand will guide me,
> your right hand will hold me fast.**'**

We are not alone. One of Jesus' names, Immanuel, means 'God with us.' If all our friends desert us, he is always there. Sometimes it's hard to believe that — Jesus' disciples could hardly believe it.

The last time the disciples saw Jesus, they were huddled together in enormous pain and grief. They thought their beloved friend and master was leaving them forever. But Jesus comforted them. 'Surely I am with you always, to the very end of the age.'

If you allow Jesus into your life, that promise is

for you. He will come to you in the middle of the night when you awaken, sweaty and afraid. Or when a feeling of loneliness steals over you in the midst of a crowd. Or when you have just been given your latest blood-test results. You are not alone. Jesus is with you.

Jesus also promises us peace. Since AIDS has entered our lives, it seems as if the last thing we have in our hearts is peace. We are troubled. We are anxious. We are afraid. Jesus' disciples felt the same way when he said he was leaving.

They were upset. They were horrified. They were not feeling peaceful. And yet Jesus promised them peace.

'Peace I leave with you; my peace I give you. I do not give to you as the world gives. Do not let your hearts be troubled and do not be afraid.'

Many of us know about the peace that the world gives. Some have tried to find it through compulsive sex, drugs, alcohol, material things. This kind of peace is temporary and ultimately destructive.

The peace that Jesus offers is *his* peace — a divine peace, an inward quiet that no person, place or virus is able to destroy. It is ours for the asking.

'I had asked God into my life long before I was diagnosed with AIDS. After my diagnosis, some of my friends wondered how I could still believe in God. But God's peace and love are even more evident to me now. I am not saying that I never get scared or lonely. I guess most important is

that I know Jesus is right there with me and suffering with me. Sometimes my heart cries out in a language that only God can hear. So my friends are not able to hear those things. But I know that God hears me.'

7
Balance

'My spiritual life doesn't seem that important because all my energy is put into taking my medications, eating right, resting, and visiting my doctor.'

To deny our spiritual selves is to get out of balance. We are not only physical beings. We are also spiritual, emotional and intellectual beings. To be whole people, we need to pay attention to our whole selves.

When you are diagnosed as HIV-positive, it's easy to think of nothing but how your body feels. It's easy to let your life revolve around temperatures, lab results and searching for miracle cures. As you frantically race around, anxiety and fears can build up.

To find peace, we need to slow down and take time for our inner selves. We need to recognize our feelings and be open with our fears. We need to be still and listen for God's voice speaking to our hearts.

When we consciously spend time in God's presence, we automatically center ourselves. It is as if we are in the eye of a hurricane. While the storm rages around us, we are peaceful and calm in the center.

There is never any reason to hurry before God. The psalmist calls God a rock. A rock is solid, strong, centered. What could be less frantic than a rock?

You may feel that because you are HIV-positive, you have to race through life, doing everything and seeing everyone. But a good life does not mean having *more* life experiences, but experiencing life more *fully*. Quality, not quantity.

We can choose to make every moment count. We can notice the shadow of leaves on the sidewalk, the sounds of birds overhead, the smell of coffee, flowers, an old leather jacket.

We can learn to really *be* with people. Not hastily *doing* but simply *being*. Listening — not thinking of our next word, but concentrating fully on the other person. Hearing every word. Hearing between the words.

Life is more than medicine and hospitals. When all we think about is our physical state, we become imbalanced. No wonder some people feel as if they are about to tip over.

Our hearts and minds and spirits get as hungry as our bodies. They need feeding too. We feed our inner selves through prayer, meditation, reading the Bible. To be whole people, we need to take care of our whole selves.

> *'The minute I found out I had AIDS, I began living my life at ninety miles per hour. I was diagnosed in December and, on Christmas Day, I went to* **three** *different Christmas dinners. I wanted to see everyone and do everything. But*

I ended up feeling exhausted and not even remembering what happened at those three dinners. So I slowed down a bit. But then if I had a day when I was feeling ill, I would get scared and anxious and start running around all over again. I'd see new doctors and go to different clinics.

'One day on the way home from a doctor's appointment, I stopped at a red light right next to a church. There was one of those boards that they invariably have in front of churches. On it were the words, "Be still and know that I am God." I don't know exactly why, but I was stunned. Be still? It sounded like a revolutionary concept to me.

'When I got home I looked up that verse in the Bible and then just sat there — being still. A tremendous sense of peace came over me. Ever since then, I spend at least an hour a day just sitting and meditating or praying. I'm not sure what to call it. I've realized that life is more than doctors, clinics and an active social life.'

8

Relationships

'AIDS has made me see that the most important things in my life are my relationships with others. That gives me a lot of joy, but also a lot of pain, since some of my relationships are broken.'

In the same way that God reaches out in love to us, we can reach out to other people. It may feel impossible to do this. We may be so bitter, hurt and angry with someone that we can't imagine reaching out to them.

What can we do when it feels impossible to forgive? Identifying our feelings is the first step. When we try to deny anger or hurt, the feelings get stuffed down deep inside us, but they don't disappear. Instead they keep us from loving God, ourselves and others.

Finding someone to talk with is helpful. A caring friend can help us sort out our feelings and express them. Then, when we reach out, we can do so cleanly and directly, without having to make our way through a mess of emotions.

We can ask God to heal our hearts and give us the love, courage and strength to reach out. We can ask God to help us love ourselves so that our self-esteem is not dependent on the opinions and actions of other people.

What if our attempts to mend relationships are rejected? We can't be responsible for another person's reaction, but we can accept it. Sometimes people need time to heal their own wounds and aren't yet ready to be reconciled. Our responsibility is to build a bridge halfway and then hope others build their part, thus closing the gap.

> *'I have always felt a deep bitterness toward my parents and my ex-husband. I thought I could ignore these feelings and just get on with my life since I had my children and my friends. Then I found out I had AIDS and suddenly it seemed vitally important that I mend those relationships — or at least make an effort.*
>
> *'It turned out that time had healed a lot of the wounds between my parents and me. We were able to talk about the past and plan for the future. We were even able to grieve together.*
>
> *'Things did not work as well with my ex-husband. He is still angry and refuses to talk. As I reached out, my vision cleared and I saw him as the wounded man he really is. Because I could see him this way, I did not stay angry with him. Because I know he is hurting, I have the patience to wait until he is ready to talk.'*

9

Love

'All my life people have been telling me to do this and do that — and then they'll love me. I've tried to change myself to please everyone. Do I have to be a better person to experience God's love, or does God really love me just the way I am?'

God loves and accepts us just as we are. We don't have to do anything to earn God's love. Some of us have spent most of our lives trying to earn love, and we can't imagine that it could be any other way. We've tried to make more money, get better grades, build a better body — all to make ourselves more 'lovable.' But none of that is necessary with God.

God loves us — right now — simply for who we are. No entrance requirements. No fees. No questions asked.

There is no expiration date on God's love. God's love endures *forever*.

To see God's love in action, we can look at the

life of Jesus. He loved all people. He loved people who were considered outcasts by society.

He dined with cheats and prostitutes. He talked to little children. He touched lepers.

AIDS has caused many to feel like modern-day lepers — untouchable and cast out. But we are never cast out by God. Our wounded hearts are touched by God's healing love.

God's love is not some abstract theological concept. God's love is real. It comes in many different packages.

God's love comes in a hug or a phone call from a friend. It comes in a meal brought by a neighbor. God's love comes in a good laugh, or a good cry. It comes in the smile of a stranger.

And in those moments when we feel as if we have no more tears to shed or screams to scream, the love of God enfolds us like warm, strong arms.

God's love has an eternal guarantee and it is returnable. We can give that love back to God, to our neighbors and to ourselves. It never decreases, but increases with use.

'I am embarrassed to say this, but the truth is that I never felt loved. I went to classy schools and wore fancy clothes, but I was always trying to be someone I really wasn't. I hated science, but I endured four years of pre-med because my parents wanted me to be a doctor.

'I finally stopped trying to please them when I moved away. But I had become a chameleon — I could change into anybody you wanted me to be.

'Because of AIDS two things have happened for me: one, I am physically too tired to keep changing all the time, and two, I see how senseless it really is. After my diagnosis I began exploring my spirituality and realized that God loves me just the way I am. Knowing that gave me the courage to love myself — just the way I am.'

10
Healing

'I think a lot about healing. I want to be healed but I'm not sure if I'm supposed to find a doctor to do it, heal myself, or let God do it.'

Healing is not the same as curing. *Curing* means taking away a physical illness. *Healing* is much more. It is a drawing together of the heart, mind and body. It is a return to wholeness.

Sometimes it is our hearts which need to be healed. Perhaps we have wounds there filled with bitterness, anger, hatred and fear. In order for our hearts to be healed, we must open them to care and love from others and ourselves.

At first this may be difficult, especially if we have been careful about hiding our hurt. So we need to gently name the hurt and brokenness in our hearts. Then we can talk about it — to ourselves, to our friends, to God.

It is important to be gentle with ourselves. There is no timetable, no standard by which to measure healing.

We need to allow ourselves to heal in our way, at our own pace. It is a process, not a one-shot cure.

A healed heart is open. It does not criticize. It meets others with acceptance and love. It knows that other people are different, not 'bad,' 'stupid' or 'weird.' A healed heart meets itself with love.

Our minds may need healing too. Suspicion, mistrust and fear can make our minds narrow and intolerant. Our thoughts can become negative, hurtful and violent. We see things only in black and white. A healed mind, like a healed heart, is open. A healed mind considers all sides, sees alternatives, realizes that life can be 'both/and,' not simply 'either/or.'

Since wholeness includes the physical body, each person with AIDS needs to seek treatment and work with a doctor. This means following instructions for medication, diet and rest. This may sound obvious, but if you have not really accepted the diagnosis, you may conveniently 'forget' about your medications or diet. You somehow think that if you disregard the prescriptions for your disease, then you don't have the disease.

Although it is important to follow your doctor's instructions, it is equally important to realize that *you* have some choices. You can be honest, ask questions, request information. You can take some responsibility for the management of your disease. You are just as important as your doctor in dealing with AIDS.

Dr. Albert Schweitzer said that most patients do not know that they carry their own doctor around inside them. Physicians are at their best, he said, when they give the doctor who resides within each patient a chance to go to work.

How many of us really know the 'doctor within'? Most of us live in our heads and don't know how to listen to our hearts anymore — until we are forced to. Until now. Until we realize that all the brilliant thinking in the world is not the answer. Healing includes an opening of the heart.

The gospel writer Luke tells of a woman who had been bleeding for twelve years. No one could heal her. And yet, immediately after she touched the edge of Jesus' cloak, her bleeding stopped. The power of Jesus? The opening of the woman's heart? Or both?

Jesus said, 'Someone touched me; I know that power has gone out from me.' Then he turned to the woman and said, 'Daughter, your faith has healed you. Go in peace.' His power, her faith.

Physical healing might also mean an awareness and new love for our bodies. Perhaps we once regarded our bodies simply as vehicles or pleasure centers. Now we see that our bodies are not separate from our selves. Learning to care for our bodies thoughtfully and gently can be a return to wholeness.

Our hearts, minds and bodies are not three separated parts of us. They are connected and intermeshed. Often, healing in one place results in healing in another. When we are healing in all places, then we are returning to complete wholeness.

'At first I threw my body at my doctor and said, "Do whatever you have to do." I didn't want to take any responsibility for my own healing. But then I started attending an AIDS support group. They all seemed to know so much about

different treatments and medications. They were even making suggestions to their doctors. People were talking about visualizing God's healing love filling their bodies and how their spirits were being healed, even though physically they weren't doing too well.

'*One guy who died seemed happier and more at peace with himself than when he was healthy! This was the first time I realized that death is not a failure.*'

11

Death

'I don't want to hear about death. I don't want to talk about death. I want to be as positive as possible.'

What does it mean if you seem to be getting worse, instead of better? Does it mean you are not trying hard enough? Or that your doctors are ineffective? Or that God doesn't care?

When the woman in the gospel story touched Jesus' robe, she was healed into life. Unlike her, some of us will be healed into death.

When we realize that healing, a return to wholeness, can include death, we can see that death is no longer the enemy. Death is a part of life.

There is a fine line between being positive and denying reality. For living and healing, it is important to develop a positive attitude. It is also important to face death.

Denying death takes a lot of energy. You have to work hard at *not* thinking about death. Every time you have your blood drawn, swallow a pill, look in the mirror, you have to face death. Think how much energy it takes to deny it!

But how can we face death and go on with our lives? Doesn't accepting death mean that we have given up living? Absolutely not. Is a good book or film any less enjoyable because we know it is going to end?

It is the same way with life — for all of us. Because whether we have AIDS or not, we are all going to die. Being HIV-positive makes you face that reality sooner.

When we face death, we then free up our energy. Instead of using our energy to deny death, we can use that energy to live. We can use that energy to change. We can use that energy to love.

Talking about death and trying to understand death can take the fear out of it. If we turn on a light in a dark room, suddenly all the shadows disappear.

In the Bible, Jesus is described as the true light that gives light to every person who comes into the world. Jesus himself said, 'I am the light of the world. Whoever follows me will never walk in darkness, but will have the light of life.'

By his death and resurrection, Jesus conquered death. Death no longer holds nameless terrors for people who live in Jesus' light.

We don't have to wait until we're dying to turn and face the light. We can turn our attention to God and ask for the light right now. By opening our hearts to Christ, we can live in the light and share in Christ's victory over death.

Death means the end of this life, but not the end of all life. For all who open their hearts to Christ, there is the promise of resurrection and renewal — new health and strength — not only for us, but also for the earth. Here is an image of restoration written by the prophet Isaiah:

'You will go out in joy
    and be led forth in peace;
the mountains and hills
    will burst into song before you,
and all the trees of the field
    will clap their hands.
Instead of the thornbush will grow the pine tree,
    and instead of briers the myrtle will grow.'

'It seems bizarre — now that I know I have AIDS, I actually feel more whole than I ever did before. I am sure it is because I have asked the Light into my life, and I have been forced to face death. For me that meant looking at areas of my life that I have always put on hold.

'Now I just don't have that much time to waste. Death is not frightening to me since I feel that I have made peace with myself. In fact, I think that death is not the end of the journey. It is like going to Kansas City on your way to somewhere else. Kansas City is no big deal; it's the rest of the journey that's important. Unfortunately, no one has come back from death (as they have from Kansas City) to tell us what it is like. So we make a big deal out of it.'

12

Pain

'I'm not afraid of death as much as I am afraid of dying. The actual process of dying scares me. I am afraid of pain.'

No one can say for sure whether death will be painful or not. But we do know that pain is increased when we are afraid and resistant. Women in labor are encouraged to breathe deeply and consciously relax their muscles to help them deal with the pain.

As one new mother explained, 'There is a difference between suffering and pain. Suffering is when I resist the pain. But when I accept the pain and relax and just let it be, then I am not suffering. Labor pains, of course, produce something beautiful — a child. But I think most physical pain, if we don't resist it, can produce something beautiful in us.'

We don't want to deny, romanticize or glorify pain. Accepting pain doesn't mean liking it or being quiet about it. It means allowing the pain to break down the old in us so that we may discover the new. It means letting the pain be a mirror for us to see the places in our lives that have become small and narrow. It means seeing the pain decrease the distance between our hearts and minds.

Pain can be like a sharp knife. It slices through years of pretension, hiding and fakery to reveal our true selves. Selves that we kept from unfolding. Selves that we need to love and accept.

Seen in this way, pain can indeed give birth to a new being.

'Not being an athletic person, I always hated that slogan, "No pain, no gain." I spent most of my life avoiding any kind of pain. AIDS has made me get to know pain in a new way. Some of the medicine I was on at first made me feel sicker than ever. At that point I learned that when I tensed up, or tried to distract myself, my pain actually seemed worse. It is paradoxical, but the more I just allowed myself to be in the pain, look it right in the eye, the less intense it became. I can't explain how this works — I can only tell you that it does.

'Because of being with the pain, I have seen sides of myself that I had never seen before. Sides that I like! Sides that I admire! I wish I could have seen these sides some other way — I don't recommend going out and contracting AIDS so you can find yourself. Anyway, I hate to admit it, but now I understand and agree with "No pain, no gain."'

13

Grief

'I have already lost many of my friends to AIDS. And now I must deal with my own death. I am overwhelmed by grief. I can think of nothing else.'

Grief is demanding. If we don't pay attention to it, it will force itself on us until we can think, do and feel nothing else. So we need to make time for tears. We need to make time to cry alone and cry together.

Grief is about loss. AIDS is about the loss of your friends, the loss of your health. In your grief you search for what is lost. Sometimes you go to the places your friends used to go. Sometimes you look at photographs of yourself when you were strong and healthy.

It is all right to search for what is lost. When we recognize that the loss can never be regained, our grieving changes. Then we often seem to find what we have been looking for. We may feel the presence of our friends in ways that are stronger than if they were still alive.

You may give up the search for your former physical health and instead find a self you have never known. A self you never had time to nurture and love. So in the midst of your grief, you may be surprised to find joy. But this won't happen if you ignore your grief.

Grief is unpredictable. Just when we think we're feeling better, a song, a word, a picture will remind us of our loss. Then it is as if we have been hit by a tidal wave when we weren't looking. We are knocked face down and are breathless with pain. We struggle to get up again.

It's important that we allow ourselves to feel the pain and express it. Some of us need to talk it out — saying the same things over and over until we feel clear. Some of us need to cry it out — weeping until we run out of tears. Some of us need to scream it out — shouting and roaring until our pain subsides.

It is not a once-and-for-all situation. Grieving is about doing all or some of these things over and over again. As time goes by, we grieve with less intensity and less often, but we still grieve. We may grieve forever.

'Three of my friends died of AIDS the year before I was diagnosed. Even after a year, I knew I was still grieving. Then I found out I had AIDS. I thought I would run out of tears. Not only had I lost my friends the year before and was losing my own health, but now I was losing friends who were afraid of me. I could feel people distancing themselves from me and shutting me out of their lives. I coughed and they ran.

'That hurts more than losing friends through death. So I give myself time to grieve. I try not to

avoid it. Some days I go inward like a snail in its shell. I don't talk to people. I just allow myself to feel sad and depressed. I try to work at going through it since I know there is no way around it.

'*Other days I have to talk to anybody who will listen. Then I am much more outward in my grieving. And I do things that are life affirming — I bake bread, I plant flowers, I send notes and cards to my nieces and nephews. Most of all, I don't ignore my grief.*

'*Grief is like a new puppy. If you ignore a puppy, it will chew your shoes, tear up your house and generally wreak havoc. You must give loving attention to a puppy. It is the same with grief. If you ignore it, it will tear you up inside. So you must give your grief loving attention.*'

14
Hope

'AIDS kills everyone, so how can I have any hope? Wouldn't any hope be false hope?'

Hope is different from expectation. Expectation means that we assume something will happen. But hope means that we are open. Hope is always true. It is always real. Hope can mean that we are open to love, reconciliation, healing and all miracles.

Hope is supported by faith and love. You need to have faith in yourself, in your medical care, in God. You need to have love for yourself, for others and for God.

If your hope is fading, maybe you are relying on yourself too much and need to place your faith in God. Maybe you are not accepting yourself and need to have faith that you are loved and protected. Maybe you're just depressed.

The psalmist asks the question:

'Why are you downcast, O my soul?
  Why so disturbed within me?

Put your hope in God,
   for I will yet praise him,
my Savior and my God. *'*

Sometimes we need to remind ourselves that the source of our hope is the God who made us, loves us and offers us a new life.

It is all right to hope for miracles, but we must realize that miracles come in many forms.

Because of AIDS many have experienced miracles they never thought possible. They've cleaned up their lives, mended relationships, grown, matured, changed. Some have cast off old baggage and pursued new dreams. Others have learned to let go of the future and live in the present.

The experience of pain has been deeper than we ever imagined. And for some, out of that pain a new person has arisen. Many have found, and others regained, a faith in God, themselves and other people.

'I don't expect to be cured. Now that doesn't mean I don't want to be cured or hope to be cured. I am always hoping that there is some miracle drug right around the corner. But now I feel like this: it's OK to die of AIDS and it's OK to be cured of AIDS.

'Don't get me wrong; I am not thrilled I have AIDS. But I realize that some things have happened within me that could not have happened if I had been physically well. I mean things like a healing of my spirit, an acceptance of myself, an opening to God. So in a way

I am healed even when my T-cells are down. I would not trade this feeling for anything in the world.'

The Light of Jesus casts out our fears, gives us courage and comforts us. The Light helps us heal, grow and love. The Light helps us realize our interconnectedness and know that we are not alone.

It is never too late to ask God into our lives. It is never too late to reach out to one another. It is never too late even to love ourselves.